It's Not Just
A Theory

It's Not Just
A Theory

A Monograph Examining the Relationship
Between Behavior and Longevity—According
to Both Science and the Scriptures

MeekRaker Monograph #602

J. BARTHOLOMEW WALKER

Quadrakoff Publications Group, LLC
Wilmington, Delaware
USA

The Major Premise. . .

What is your plan to see your 150th birthday?
That's easy:
"Don't drink."
"Don't smoke."
"Don't take drugs.
"Eat right."
"Exercise."
"Do *x* and don't do *y*." (*Variables* are utilized here, because so much changes regarding what is considered to be healthy and unhealthy behaviors.)

The question was not about the plan to see your 85th birthday, but rather to see your 150th birthday. In the United States today, few see their 100th birthday much less their 150th.

And of course, even that isn't really good enough, as *living* alone is insufficient. One must also be *healthy* and *productive*.

However . . .

*Logically, the requirements
for well being of the physical
body should be such as to be
consistent with both the
nature and the requirements
of that which it is designed
to contain. It has been the
reliance on opinion on
material requirements,
while ignoring immaterial
requirements, that has
caused the Biblical human
ages to simply be non-
believable.*

It's Not Just
A Theory

Is it true?
Romans 6:22-23 (KJV) tells us:

*"But now being made free from sin,
and become servants to God,
ye have your fruit unto holiness,
and the end everlasting life.*

1

> *For the wages of sin is death;*
> *but the gift of God is eternal life*
> *through Jesus Christ our Lord."*

Here Paul is speaking of what is gained through Jesus (the) Christ.

The real question is whether or not he is lying. The fact of the matter, is that each and every person who was alive when Paul stated, (and likely actually wrote) this; including Paul; is in fact physically quite dead.

There is no possibility of prevarication here. Paul makes it quite clear that eternal life is obtained through Jesus Christ—yet there is no record of anyone at any time living eternally. The only possible known exception of course would be Jesus, (and possibly Elijah and/or Enoch); but Jesus did in fact "die" before He lived eternally. Great care is taken here to not state "ever lived eternally," for obvious reasons.

The actual Greek word translated as "life" is:

> "2222: zōē; from *2198*; *life* (lit or fig.): - life (time). Comp. *5590*."[2]

The actual Greek word translated as "death" is:

> "2288 thanatŏs; from *2348*; (prop. an adj. used as a noun) *death* (lit. or fig.): - x deadly, (be...) death."[3]

Assuming that Paul was telling the truth; clearly Paul was not speaking of *physical* life. The idea of *justification* resulting in salvation; refers not to physical life, but what many refer to as "spiritual" life. Paul is speaking of his belief of something which was made possible by He Who is: "The Anointed One," or "The Christ," or "The Messiah."

In accord with this belief, it was He, (Jesus), who provided a means by which that, or at least part of that, which is or was "breathed" into the *physical* body when *physical* life began; could return to its "spiritual" source, despite being soiled by sin. This "life" to which Paul refers, is this eternal connection to God. This represents an *immaterial* ("soul") to *immaterial* (God) connection.

But "physical life" is also a connection. That which is "*breathed*" into the physical body at birth is "connected" to the physical body as long as it, (the physical body), has this "life." When the connection begins; this is "physical birth." When the connection is severed; this is "physical death." Here this represents an *immaterial* to *material* connection. And although it seems that no one has ever maintained this connection longer than Methuselah; compared to "eternal," even Methuselah did not maintain this, (immaterial to material), connection for very long.

But what about this immaterial, ("soul"), connection to the material (physical) body?

Genesis 2:7 (KJV) tells us:

> *"And the LORD God formed man*
> *of the dust of the ground,*
> *and breathed into his nostrils*
> *the breath of life;*
> *and man became a living soul."*[4]

Here God "breathed," or in the original Hebrew:

> "5301 nâphach; a prim. root; to *puff*, in various applications..."[5]

This is the *action*, or the *means*, by which something was introduced into what would later be called "Adam's" nostrils.

What it was that God breathed or *nâphach*(ed) into what would later be called "Adam's" nostrils, was *breath*, or:

> "5397; n\u1d49shâmâh; fr. 5395; a *puff*, i.e. *wind*, angry or vital *breath*...;"[6]

And the particular type of "puff" or "wind" that was "breathed" was:

> "2416 chay; from 2421; *alive*; hence raw (flesh); fresh (plant, water, year), strong; also (as noun, espec. in the fem. sing. and masc. plur.) life (or living thing), whether lit. or fig..." [The very next word in Strong's (2417), is likewise: "chay (Chald.)" also means "*alive*" or "*life*," but here the original *Chaldean*.][7]

Here is seen a twofold process:

First, God formed the vessel utilizing matter. Then he breathed into this vessel, the *n\u1d49shâmâh*, or breath of *chay*, or life.

As a result of this "Adam" became a "*living soul*," or:

"5315 nephesh; from 5314; prop. a *breathing* creature..."[8]

[Note: Adam was *formed* from *something*. This is in contradistinction to the events in Genesis 1:27 where God *created* man. The use of the term creation means to bring into existence from *nothing*; and is a translation of the Hebrew word *bârâ'*. Here in Genesis 2:7, God is not creating from nothing; but rather is *forming* from *something*. "Formed" as opposed to "created" is a translation of an entirely different word: *yâtsar*. These are two entirely separate and distinct events, with the creation of man likely occurring many hundreds of thousands of years ago; and the formation of adam or Adam occurring less than ten thousand yeas ago. It is because of the conflation and confusion of these two events that the actual Scriptural age of the earth is in dispute with science, and believed to be less than ten thousand years old. It is beyond the scope of this monograph to litigate this, but an exhaustive explanation can be found in the first four chapters of *"Meekraker Beginnings. . ."*]

Here it is God Himself Who is bringing into existence a man in a fashion similar to the method used in "normal" human gestation and birth. With H. Sapiens, first the vessel is formed, and when completed, exits the womb. *Then and only then*, breath is drawn in by

5

the completed vessel, and it becomes a *living* or breathing physical entity. H. Sapiens even have an anatomical "insurance policy" in effect with regard to this, as the cardiac *foramen ovale,* (after birth becoming the *fossa ovale*); prevents the *premature* entrance of this breath.

One key point of this event is that here God did it Himself, without recourse, or any aid from man; i.e.; with no assistance from any of the offspring of the original *created* hosts.

The question must be asked as to what it is that is contained in this *breath*, (nᵉshâmâh); of *life*, (chay)?

It is fair to say that at least two things are contained in this "breath of life."

Firstly; would be that which is often described as *soul.* Soul is often described; erroneously, incompletely, or otherwise; as "will, intellect, and emotions." "*I am*," or a sense or knowledge of existence or "*being*," is also another way to describe soul. Soul is the immaterial and immortal portion that requires justification for reconnection to God. This "I am," is the only thing that true solipsists actually "know." It is this "soul," for which the body or vessel is designed to contain.

The *second* thing contained in this "breath of life" is the means by which the vessel sustains and maintains itself. Known as the VLF or *vital life force* by some; *Innate Intelligence* by others, or *chi* by yet others; it is this VLF that is responsible for maintaining the vessel. It is this VLF that regulates growth and healing; and can transform a ham sandwich into skin, fingernails or whatever else it; within certain limitations; deems necessary.

Since this VLF comes from God, it must then necessarily be perfect when it is "transmitted."

A quick recap of Paul's words:

> *"But now being made free from sin,*
> *and become servants to God,*
> *ye have your fruit unto holiness,*
> *and the end everlasting life.*
> *For the wages of sin is death;*
> *but the gift of God is eternal life*
> *through Jesus Christ our Lord."*

The question becomes whether or not what Paul stated could in any way apply to *physical* life.

With regard to the second verse, often; the word "penalty" is erroneously attributed to Paul, and not the word "wages;" thus making this "penalty of sin." Any such erroneous attribution, would of course change the meaning entirely.

The actual Greek word translated as "wages" is:

"3800 ŏpsōniŏn; neut. of a presumed der. of the same as 3795; *rations* for a soldier, i.e. (by extens.) his *stipend* or *pay*: - wages."[9] (It must be noted that no *reasonable* relationship between 3800 and 3795 could be found.)

7

Clearly there is an implication of the giving of what is due here, without regard to any type of penalty or reward; but rather *balance*. Wages or *ŏpsōniŏn* are paid as a matter of entitlement, and are required for that which has been performed. Wages usually represent something positive that benefits the worker, for his or her *previous* efforts that benefitted the person paying the wages.

However; in a sense, most criminal "penalties" also represent wages; but here in the *negative* sense. These "criminal" "wages" or *ŏpsōniŏn*, usually represent something negative that harms the "worker," for his or her previous act or acts of omission or commission, which resulted in injury to some party or parties. These are required in order to *balance* said act or acts of omission or commission, that resulted in injury to some party or parties.

Clearly when Paul uses ŏpsōniŏn with regard to "*sin*," he is not referring to the former positive ŏpsōniŏn; but rather the latter negative ŏpsōniŏn as contextually, said ŏpsōniŏn is "death."

It is also interesting that Paul chose ŏpsōniŏn; "no reasonable relationship," notwithstanding; that nevertheless according to Strong, refers to soldiers. This may be because according to the Father; (see Genesis 2:1 and elsewhere); all H. Sapiens are "hosts," (English), or "tsâbâ'," (Hebrew);"[10] and thus were created and designed to engage in warfare; arguably for redemption of that beyond themselves.

There is no question that engaging in certain types of "sinful" *physical* actions can result in early death. Here there is an observable relationship between these actions, and the effects of these actions on the biological vessel—suicide being a prime example. The wages or *ŏpsōniŏn* of attempted suicide; if successful; is physical death.

There is also no question that engaging in certain "*non-physical*" "actions" can have an effect on "longevity;"—either way.

Some of this can be explained in physical terms, and yet some cannot. "Stress;" as commonly understood; is considered to be a causative factor in certain types of physical ailments. Although the "stress" may be the result of physical causes; and thus the "stress" itself thus represents an *effect* of this cause; this "stress" in itself becomes a non-physical or *immaterial cause*, often with a subsequent physical or *material* result.

It matters little that the *cause* of the stress may originate in the physical, and thus be an actuality. The fact is that the "stress" itself is a *reality* and not an actuality, and thus is *subjective* in nature. The *effect* of the actual *cause* of the stress is the stress itself. But this immaterial reality of stress is now a *cause* and can have significant physical *effects* or results. And the actual cause of "stress" for one, may be a source of its opposite for another. Some cultures even celebrate physical death.

Positive experiences can work in a similar manner; but unlike stress, these can result in increased longevity and quality of life.

Today there are established "norms" as to what the "upper end" of longevity could possibly be; with few claiming these can be exceeded by any significant percentage. If it is so stipulated that the average person in the United States lives to about eighty years of age; then even a 30% change in this either way is extremely unusual—as most people live way beyond fifty six; and very few genuinely exceed one hundred and four years of age.

Methuselah lived 969 years;[11] and if a bit of math is done, it can be determined that Adam lived a minimum of 930 years. These represent increases over today's average longevity of 1211% and 1162% respectively; and thus are significant percentages of increases in longevity.

"But everyone 'knows' that this is 'mathematical hyperbole.'" Very few people today actually believe those "Bible" longevity numbers. This of course is part of the problem. There is one person who lived quite some time ago, who actually *believed* these numbers. This is a certainty, as it was he (Moses) himself, who is believed to have actually been the author initially involved in recording them.

However; in Psalms 90:8-10 (KJV), (Psalm 90 is considered to be of Mosaic authorship); where Moses is speaking to God, we are told:

"Thou hast set our iniquities before thee, our secret sins in the light of thy countenance.
For all our days are passed away in thy wrath: we spend our years as a tale that is told.
The days of our years are threescore years and ten; and if by reason of strength they be fourscore years, yet is their strength labour and sorrow;
for it is soon cut off, and we fly away."[12]

Although this may read like Shakespeare; it is not. Here Moses is noting the relationship between sin; and what he is presenting as either what he considers premature physical death, or "man's" physical death itself. And it is curious that the number of years people physically lived at the time this was written (lifespan); was between seventy and eighty—roughly about the same as today, or perhaps just a few decades ago. According to Moses, this was because: "*Thou hast set our iniquities before thee, our secret sins in the light of thy countenance. For (because) all our days are passed away in thy wrath: we spend our years as a tale that is told.*"

Moses further states how longevity is or can be increased from "threescore years and ten" (70 years); to "fourscore" (80 years); and that means is: "*by reason of strength.*"

The actual Hebrew word translated here as "strength" is:

> 1369 geᵇbûwrâh; fem. pass. part. from the same as 1368; *force* (lit. or fig.);. . ."[13]

Thus the actual stated reason for said increased longevity is in fact not *strength*, but rather *force*.

In the *incorrect* translation of *geᵇbûwrâh* as "strength;" contextually, there is a clear implication that it is the magnitude of the capability to *resist* sin that increases longevity.

Presumably, said "strength" then results in less sinful behavior. Here the active party is the "sinner." Depending simply upon both upon the magnitude of the capability to resist sin, and presumably its utilization by the otherwise sinner; here according to "The Big M," longevity can be enhanced by about 14%.

However with the *correct* translation of gᵉbûwrâh as *force*, this changes things a bit. Here the active entity *at the time* is not the sinner, but rather is a *force*. It is actually written that "by reason of *force*" that longevity is enhanced.

Thus although the "sinner" may have had much say in being the *active* party in the creation of the *original* forces by his or her behavior; here the reason for the longevity *increase*, the sinner is now the *passive* party; as he is acted upon by this gᵉbûwrâh as the recipient of a *force*. This is another example of "equal and opposite reactions;" or what is often referred to as *karma*; but here in the specific as relates to behavior (cause), and to increased longevity (effect).

This is an important distinction. The strength; (*incorrect* translation of gᵉbûwrâh); to *behave* in a proper or sinless manner is always a current or "real time" phenomenon. One cannot *currently*, (real time), sin in the past; neither can one *currently* sin in the future. Each "real time" event is when decisions are actually made. Certainly one can regret past bad decisions, or pledge to do right in the future; but ultimately the specific decisions must be made "real time;" and thus are subject to a variety of factors, including the influence of the enemy, either directly or indirectly through others. ("I know I swore never to do it again, but I really needed the money.")

But a *force*; (*correct* translation of gᵉbûwrâh); is another matter. As is always the case with "equal and opposite reactions;" i.e.; *karma*; the return force is both inevitable and unavoidable. Thus in a sense, to the extent that one's *behavior* is such that it would create forces that tend to increase longevity as Moses stated (as a *cause*); the *result* of increased longevity, (as an *effect*), is a certainty; as this increase is directly precipitated by a *force*.

But where is this "force?" In the situation cited by Moses, it seems that the force is not generally needed until 70 (seventy) years of age. So precisely where resides this particular force for the preceding "*threescore years and ten*?"

Newton's laws of inertia, F=MA and equal and opposite reactions; are usually concerned strictly with the physical. However whenever any consciousness or any "I am" is exerting free will, there is also an *immaterial* component, which is in addition to the *material* components as addressed by Newton.

Thus the actual force created is a combination of that which is produced in the material, (the action); as well as that which is produced in the immaterial, (reason for the action). [The "*Second Intermission*" of "*MeekRaker Beginnings. . .*" provides a specific and highly detailed description of this process.]

Once any action is undertaken by a conscious being, *two* actual imbalances are created. One imbalance is in the material, with another simultaneously created in the immaterial. Thus the *true*, *complete*, or *total* force, (true actuality); is a combination of both material *and* immaterial forces.

The *material* part of the force is generally balanced quickly. It takes little time for a baseball or a golf ball to move once a force is imparted to it. Irrespective of the amount of time allocated to scheming; the actual *telling* of the words of a lie; or the actual *stealing* of something; happens relatively quickly. This is the balancing of the *physical* imbalance created by the action.

However the *immaterial* component of the action behaves a bit differently. Just as F=MA applies to the material, it also applies in the immaterial; but there is substantial leeway involved in the balancing of the *immaterial* portion of the force. Whatever the magnitude of the immaterial portion of the original force, there are essentially infinite combinations for the "return" of this force. The *immaterial* "MA," or that which balances the original *immaterial* force, actually consists of two factors:

First there is the magnitude of what is returned, or the M. Then there is the timing, (how rapidly), is this return, or the A. The product of these must always equal the magnitude of the original force or "F." Thus if the immaterial force is to be balanced quickly, this represents a large value for A, or the *acceleration* of the return to the original source. However with a "quick return," the *magnitude* of what is returned must be small in order to balance the original force. Similarly; if the magnitude or "M" is to be large; then the return must be slower; (less acceleration or "A" to return to the source); in order to balance the original force. This acceleration can be extremely slow (years), if a large return is to be provided. It is God alone Who determines both the magnitude and the acceleration of these (karmic) forces directed *to the source* of the original force.

These immaterial forces reside in the immaterial as an imbalance until they intersect the material at the appropriate time, as determined by God. And God is certainly smart enough to not provide the return of forces which will increase longevity until they are necessary.

The second appearance of "*strength*," contained in: "*yet is their strength labour and sorrow; for it is soon cut off, and we fly away*;" is an entirely different word.

Here the actual Hebrew word translated as "strength" is in fact:

"7296 rôhab; from 7292; *pride*. . ."[14]

Although "*labour* (sic.)" seems to be a fair translation here, the actual Hebrew word translated as "*sorrow*" is:

"205 'âven; from an unused root perh. mean. prop. to *pant* (hence to *exert* oneself, usually in vain; to *come* to *naught*) strictly *nothingness*; also *trouble*, *vanity*, *wickedness*; spec. an *idol*. . ."[15]

Thus a better translation would be: "Nevertheless in their *pride, labor,* and *nothingness;* because it is soon cut off, and we fly away;"

Moses himself lived to only one hundred and twenty years of age; but was in excellent physical condition when he died.[16]

Assuming Moses wrote Psalms 90 while he was still alive, and this represents a 50% increase over the "fourscore" stated here in Psalms 90; it is far from some the life spans of others that Moses had written about.

Was Moses a sinner? It is reasonably clear that it was not because the land that God had promised Abraham,

Isaac, and Jacob was not *good* enough for Moses; that he was permitted only to see it.

But back to Paul's statement in Romans 6:22-23: "*But now being made free from sin, and become servants to God, ye have your fruit unto holiness, and the end everlasting life. For the wages of sin is death; but the gift of God is eternal life through Jesus Christ our Lord.*"

The actual Greek word translated as "free" is:

> "*1659* ĕlĕuthĕrŏō; from *1658*; to *liberate*, i.e. (fig.) to *exempt* (from mor., cer. or mortal liability): - deliver, make free."[17]

Thus this "*free from*" or *ĕlĕuthĕrŏō*, refers to some type of liberation or exemption from sin. This refers to a *binary* with respect to *immaterial* or *spiritual* life or "connection;" as it is the presence of *any* sin and not the quantity or magnitude of sin that precludes eternal connection to God.

Being "*free from sin*" refers to justification; rendering man "just as though he never sinned." This is why the characteristics of man's sin can become irrelevant *immaterially,* with respect to that eternal connection. This justification by Jesus prevents "spiritual" death or disconnection, as the result of or from any and all sin.

But being free from or *ĕlĕuthĕrŏō* from sin, is not the same as being "sin free."

Although man is ĕlĕuthĕrŏō from the contamination of sin *immaterially* with respect to justification with regard to *future* immaterial life; there has not been any type of justification provided for the *material* effects of sin. Materially, the "here and now" *material* wages of sin are still "physical death."

It cannot be overemphasized that *materially* here means not only the relatively quick *direct* material results of sin; but also the *indirect* material effect of sin, by the ultimate *material* return of manifestations (karma), as the result of the imbalances created in the *immaterial*.

This is likely why Jesus "gave up His Spirit" on the cross—He had no alternative. Being sin free, likely He simply could not die any other way. No sin—then no wages of sin or physical death. Death by crucifixion generally took 2-3 days, but Jesus gave up his life the same day the crucifixion began. This is why Pilate was surprised that Jesus was "dead already." Thus; contrary to the common belief of some, Jesus was not *killed*. This act, (killing), requires a third party to "*take*" Jesus' life; as opposed to how the Scriptures read in that He *gave* His life.

If this is so stipulated, then it seems that there is a relationship between sin and physical death; in that without sin there can be no physical death; and with sin physical death at some point in time is a certainty.

Proverbs 9:10-11 tells us:

"The fear of the LORD is the
beginning of wisdom:
and the knowledge of the
holy is understanding.
For by me thy days shall be
multiplied, and the years of thy
life shall be increased."[8]

As is generally the case, the word "*fear*" here in this context, should have been translated as "reverence."

The actual Hebrew word is:

> "3374 yir'âh; fem. of 3373; *fear* (also used as infin.); mor. *reverence*: - x dreadful, x exceedingly, fear (-fulness).[19]

Here we are told that it is possible to increase the years of one's life by beginning *wisdom*, and obtaining *understanding*. This will happen by Him, ("*Me*").

How does this happen? This happens by altering behavior from that which is *not* known or understood—perceiving some short term gain as a singular entity; to that which *is* understood. Once the long term results, (even outside of longevity), of upright behavior are known and understood; the result is less sin. This "by Him" will necessarily multiply days and increased years. It is not a matter of "*strength*," but simply a matter of *forces*.

Exodus 20:12 tells us:

> "Honour thy father and thy mother:
> that thy days may be long upon the land
> which the LORD thy God giveth thee."[20]

Here again we are told of the relationship between behavior and longevity. The inclusion of "*upon the land which the Lord thy God giveth thee;*" is provided to be certain that it is understood that this refers to *physical* life.

It could be fair to consider old age and death as a sub-clinical disease. It would be more accurate to say that it is a pandemic sub-clinical disease which is always fatal; (except for one, or possibly as many as three: Jesus, and possibly Elijah and/or Enoch). Of course the concept that a "sub-clinical disease" that "everyone has which is always fatal;" seems absurd.

It would be *"fair-er;"* to consider old age and/or death, as a *clinical* disease, which remains unrecognized as such because of its ubiquitous nature. Since everyone ultimately acquires this disease; it is not considered as a disease, except in rare instances such as *progeria*.

Although *immaterially*, as little as even one sin guarantees *spiritual* death that can only be remedied by justification; the *amount* of sin is irrelevant with respect to justification.

With *physical* death, it seems that although even one sin results in the onset of the disease; the "prognosis" can vary greatly—*if longevity and health are the prime considerations*. These variations in longevity and health are the result of the *amount* of sin.

Sin is much more like a slow acting poison, administered over a long period of time; which accumulates in the system, and ultimately results in "physical death." The less sin administered; the greater amount of time before the onset of death. However; even with only one administration, *physical death becomes a certainty*. It would just take much longer to manifest.

But the onset and duration of "normal" old age and subsequent physical death is rather peculiar. There are various opinions regarding when this transition occurs;

many believing that thirty three years of age is the average point of transition. Some may believe that this point is where catabolism, (breaking down), begins to overtake anabolism, (building up). There are also large variations in the outward physical manifestations of this disease.

So the actual cause of this unrecognized disease remains unknown. Since the morbidity and mortality is 100%, it is believed that the causative factor of this unrecognized disease must simply be the presence of life—that being both a prerequisite and a common factor. If one is alive; then barring any trauma, there must necessarily still be physical death at some point; this merely being a "fact of life."

But while it is most certainly true and cannot be argued, that all who are living are in fact living; there is also another *activity* that currently all commonly engage in; and that other activity is *sin*. Being physically alive is a binary, but sinning; although another ultimate certainty; is much more varied. Since all men sin, and the wages of sin is death; ultimately all "H. Sapiens" soldiers obtain their *ŏpsōniŏn* or "rations, stipend, or pay."

If a *recognized* clinical disease is diagnosed; then this disease state is recognized, and appropriate treatment can be instituted.

But if an *unrecognized* pandemic disease is in progress, along with the belief that the signs and symptoms are not because of any *disease*, but rather are because of *design*; then nothing *will* be done, because it is believed that there is nothing that *needs* to be done, or *can* be done.

In the "miracles" of the Bible, where diseased persons were healed by Jesus and others; this generally represented the "casting out" of the entity that was responsible for the malady. (To be accurate; usually this was actually a matter of authority, and not supernatural power; except in those cases where gross visible physical changes were immediate.) In each of these cases, these were recognizable, (physical or mental), diseases.

According to the testimony; the demonic infiltration had reached the level where it (or they), was or were, capable of causing sufficient disruption, as to produce the signs and symptoms of disease. Leprosy, blood disorders, withered hands and the like, were not considered a normal "part of life." These had passed the threshold for clinical disease.

However; merely because interfering entities have not succeeded in sufficient disruptions as to produce clinical signs and symptoms indicative of *recognized* or *recognizable* disease; this does not mean that there are no disruptions that are taking place.

"Everyone dies from something." This "one" is unfortunately true. If the position is taken that old age and subsequent physical death is by design; barring clinical disease, trauma, etc.; then all die by design. But if the position is taken that physical death is not by design; then all "natural" death, (barring trauma); is in fact by some type of *disease*; irrespective of how long "old age" takes to be fatal.

If the "*wages of sin is death*;" whether "spiritual" death or "physical" death; then there is a clear implication that without sin, there would be no death. Surely this is so in the sense of "spiritual" death. Of

21

what use would justification be for one who never sinned? The problem is that this only happened once. There is only that one man who never sinned; yet he still died. It is true that He died; but again it is also true that neither anyone nor anything killed Him. He *chose* to give up the immaterial/material connection, and the record is clear on this. Attempts were made to kill Him and each failed. He told His disciples that no man could kill him; and again, the account of this willful severing of the immaterial/material connection by Him is recorded.

This leads to an interesting dilemma: Had Jesus *not chosen* to sever that immaterial/material connection; then it is arguable that He would have lived forever. Since He had never sinned, there were no wages, and physical death would not have been possible.

However; had He chosen to not sever that immaterial/material connection; this itself would have been a sinful act, as this was one of the main reasons for His physical existence. Attacks about this decision, (to go through with it); formed the basis for what happened at Gethsemane.

"The years have been kind to him;" is an expression which in a sense is antithetical to Paul's wisdom. Here there is an unusual condition under observation; with attribution to this anomaly being an unspecified, but relatively long duration of time. The truth is likely that "he had been kind to the years;" in the sense of working a "low paying" job in the sin department. Here at least there is a reasonable cause for the observed effect.

————————————

The facts are that aging is a disease which violates biological law; and biological law violates non-biological law. What could this mean, and does this make any degree of sense?

Non-biological law generally *decreases* the level of organization as a function of time. Diffusion, osmosis, radioactive decay; all result in lower levels of organization and higher levels of entropy. Geographical changes over time; result in lower levels of organization. The proper maintenance of a home; is a means to minimize and reverse these disorganizing forces. Fences must be painted; as a painted fence represents a much higher level of organization, which natural forces will over time disorganize. The list goes on.

But biological laws result in *higher* levels of organization. The changes that occur in a developing embryo seem miraculous. The human body can transform relatively low levels of matter such as oxygen, water and simple organic compounds into levels of organization so complex, that even today they are barely understood. The structure of the nervous system; as well as the chemicals used in its functioning; can "automatically" be made or modified from much less organized forms of matter such as fruits, vegetables, and hunks of animal muscle. The same can be said of the remainder of the human structure.

To suggest that this biological process, (maintaining the vessel or body), by design and thus on its own, somehow begins to fail at some point in time; *without* any interfering factors; represents an "explanation" which is based upon observation only. In order for this to be true, then this Vital Life Force, Innate

Intelligence, or chi, must change, (begin to fail), as a matter of *intentional* and *deliberate* design; i.e.; "God's will." [It should be asked which specific *subsets* of that *set* known as "God," contain imperfection?]

The alternative explanation being; that it is caused by an *interfering* factor, to which no one currently alive has 100% immunity; and thus *all* eventually will contract this disease.

Any empirically based assumption(s) that it is the *organizing* force (VLF) which fails by design; does not in any way mean that this assumption is correct. Neither does it mean that another causative factor does not exist.

In the physical science of electricity, one of the most fundamental laws is Ohm's Law; expressed as $E = IR$.

Here E is **E**lectromotive force or voltage; I is the current, flow of electrons or **I**ntensity; and R is the **R**esistance to that flow.

This law describes the relationship of the simple circuit. In order for current to flow, there must be: a current or movement of electrons; a force driving that current; and a load through which to drive it.

As stated in this law, the larger the driving force (E), the greater the amount of electron flow (I), through a given resistance or load (R); and the greater this resistance (R), the lesser amount of electron flow (I) for a given force (E). [Step on a garden hose and less water flows, unless the pressure is increased.]

Ohm's law is a *material* law; and like all material laws, there is a corresponding law in the *immaterial* from which it came. One example of this law in the immaterial; relates to the intentions and actions of the enemy to supplant that which is in, or is of the image and likeness of God; with that which is of him—that is; that which is not of God but is of the *enemy*.

That which is of him, (the enemy), and not of Him; is analogous to the current. The enemy needs to get his current to flow into the hosts (H. Sapiens). As in an electrical circuit, once the current gets into the hosts; then changes begin.

The enemy does this in two very basic ways with respect to this same E = IR law; with each method attempting to use forces, but with different tactical; (but the same strategic); intentions.

Firstly; he does this by the utilization of forces against the hosts that are analogous to voltage. He "cranks up" this voltage in order to get current to flow from him to the hosts. Much "actionable intelligence" can be gained by carefully observing the nature of these "voltage increases." This is because unlike voltage, there is a *subjective* component. What would be low voltage to one host, can be the same as high voltage to another; and vice versa. (This can often be the reason for what seems to be pettiness.) These forces are custom designed to produce the maximum voltage, (and ultimately maximum current flow); *for that particular host*; and thus there is much intelligence that can be obtained by the design and timing of the attack—but it also must be remembered that the enemy is not always correct.

However; just as in Ohm's law, in order for this to work; there must be the load, and that load of course is the host. But being made in the image and likeness of God; that load (host) is not a particularly good *conductor* for the enemy's "current." This necessarily means that the host *is* a particularly good *resistor*. In order to maximize the current flow for a given voltage, the enemy will also attempt to lower the host's *resistance*. Here also much "actionable intelligence" can be gained by carefully observing the nature of these attempts at lowering resistance; as the enemy will attack those areas he or it perceives as weak. But again, it must be remembered that the enemy is not always correct.

Job 1:10 tells us:

> *"Hast not thou made an hedge about him,*
> *and about his house,*
> *and about all that he hath on every side?*
> *thou hast blessed the work of his*
> *hands, and his substance is*
> *increased in the land."*[21]

Here Satan is complaining to God that He has "*made an* (sic.) *hedge*" around Job. This "hedge" results in increased resistance. And according to Ohm's law, increased resistance means less current flow, for a given voltage. Satan is essentially complaining here that the resistance is way too high, and he cannot get significant current to flow into Job. But he admits here that God is the one who "made" this hedge.

This "hedge" is actually:

> "7753 sûwk a prim. root; to *entwine*, i.e. *shut* in (for formation, protection or restraint):- fence, (make an) hedge (up)."[22]

This may seem unrelated at first, but is in fact quite relevant:

When God refers to "keeping" His commandments in Exodus 20, most believe that this "keep" or "keeping" means *obey*.

Here in Exodus the actual Hebrew word is:

> "8104: shâmar; A prim. root; prop. to *hedge* about (as with thorns), i.e. *guard*; gen. to *protect*, *attend to*, etc.: - beware, be circumspect, take heed (to self), keep (-er, self), mark, look narrowly, observe, preserve, regard, reserve, save (self), sure, (that lay) wait (for), watch (-man)."[23] [See MeekRaker Monograph #601 "*Shâmar to Sharia*"]

Thus God is not talking about *obedience*; but *protecting* His commandments with an (allegorical) "hedge." To the extent that this "hedge" is built; this also increases the host's resistance, thus making the enemy's current flow to the host difficult. This is similar to the hedge around Job; but here this "hedge" or the act of *shâmar* must be *chosen* to be made by *man*.

A fair argument can be made that in a sense, this "God made" "hedge" or *sûwk* in the case of Job, is or was primarily for the *material*; and the "man made" "hedge" or *shâmar* is for the *immaterial*. It could further be argued that this "God made" hedge varies with *action*; and the "man made" hedge varies with *thoughts*.

As this "hedgeogenic" resistance increases, either less current will flow; or the enemy must somehow "crank up" the voltage. And there are limits; albeit sometimes changeable; to the "voltages" available to him.

What about the hosts not merely maximizing the *resistance*, but also affecting the *voltage* applied by the enemy?

Paul told us how to do the former, in Ephesians 6:10-17. However unbeknownst to many, he also told us how to do the latter; but since it is a short phrase which appears at the end of a lengthy passage concerning numerous *defensive* measures, it generally goes unnoticed. What is important is that when this offensive measure is utilized; and this *cannot* be overemphasized; *it should never be combined with anything that is of the enemy*.

Ephesians 6:17 tells us:

"And take the helmet of salvation,
and the sword of the Spirit,
which is the word of God:"[24]

Tucked in here at the very end of a long list of defensive, (increasing resistance), measures in all of the verses preceding verse 17, and beginning here in verse 17 after the second "and;" something rather interesting appears. In fact; therein lies a "bomb." And it is a rather interesting and quite powerful "bomb;"—the same representing the provision of a key instruction:

> *"(take) the sword of*
> *the Spirit, which is the*
> *word of God."*

This instruction is the only *offensive,* (voltage lowering), instruction given in these famous, (Ephesians 6:10-17), verses.

What does "(take) *the sword of the Spirit, which is the word of God*" actually mean?

The actual Greek word translated as "sword" is:

> "*3162* machaira; prob. fem. of a presumed der. of *3163*; a *knife*, i.e. *dirk*; fig. *war*, judicial *punishment*: - sword."[25]

As can be seen, the translation as "sword" is misleading. A dirk is not a sword. "Knife" or "Dagger" would be a better translation. These are designed for "up close and personal" combat. This is important because this, (close up and tailor made), is precisely how the enemy attacks.

The "figurative" meaning should also be noted—that of "judicial punishment." There is an old saying: "Don't stick your head in the boxing ring if you don't want to get punched." It is the enemy who chooses to institute an attack. If the result is encountering a counterattack with a dirk, and he/it leaves a bit "bloodied;" then he or it deserved it. But again, this should never be combined with anything that is of the enemy such as anger, hatred, etc. It is *justice*, ("judicial punishment"); and not *vengeance*, that should be sought. If that which is of the enemy is *at any time* utilized, this can then easily be utilized by the enemy as a foothold.

The actual Greek word translated as "spirit" is:

> "*4151* pnĕuma; from *4154*; a *current* of air, i.e. *breath* (*blast*) or a *breeze*; by anal. or fig. a *spirit*, i.e. (human) the rational *soul*, (by impl.) *vital principle*, mental *disposition* etc..."[26]

Thus; "the knife of the soul" is a better translation. And precisely what is this "knife of the soul?"

It is the "*word of God.*" What is this "word," and why is it a machaira or "knife?"

The actual Greek "word" translated here in Ephesians as "word" is:

> "*4487* rhēma; from *4483*; an *utterance* (individ., collect. or spec.); by impl. a *matter* or *topic* (espec. of narration, command or dispute); with a neg. *naught* whatever..."[27]

John 1:1 tells us:

> "*In the beginning was the Word,*
> *and the Word was with God,*
> *and the Word was God.*"[28]

However the actual Greek word translated three times here in John as "word," is not *rhēma*, but rather:

> "3056 lŏgŏs; from 3004; something *said* (including the *thought*); by impl. a *topic* (subject of discourse), also *reasoning* (the mental faculty) or *motive*; by extens. a *computation*; spec. (with the art. In John) the Divine *Expression* (i.e. *Christ*)..."[29]

So it must be asked what the difference is between these two Greek words, each translated as "word?" The same being *rhēma* and *lŏgŏs*; and furthermore, why it was *rhēma* that was used in *Ephesians*; but it was *lŏgŏs* that was used in *John*?

Paul was giving us instructions for *future* behavior; and John was recollecting *past* events. Thus *rhēma*; meaning an *utterance*, refers to what God *is* or *will be* saying "real time." *Lŏgŏs* refers to what God has or had already "said."

Assuming Moses actually wrote early Genesis, what he recorded was the *rhēma* he was receiving "real time" from God; as he was not physically alive when those events in early Genesis transpired. In fact it seems no one was. (This process is what is referred to as *retrophesy* in "*MeekRaker Beginnings...*") Once it was recorded, however, and not being received "real time;" it then became *lŏgŏs*. The *means* of said recording; e.g.; oral memorization, long continuous scrolls, or today's Bible format; changes nothing with regard to this.

Thus this *rhēma* in "*word of God*," refers primarily to what God *will be* uttering "real time;" and represents the "knife" portion of this "knife of the soul." But this is not to say that in the absence of the reception of any rhēma, that lŏgŏs cannot be utilized just as Jesus did when the enemy attacked Him. It must be remembered that the enemy "ran away" after this particular event.[30]

Paul's use of *rhēma*, and not *lŏgŏs*, indicates a *preference*, but does not necessarily represent an absolute. Again, Jesus seems to have done pretty well with the: "It is written. . ." It is not clear that any *Greek* word exists, that includes both *rhēma* and *lŏgŏs*.

Thus when attacking the enemy with the "knife of the soul," *rhēma* is preferred; but *lŏgŏs* is also an option. It must be noted that both contain that which is of God; and that neither *original* verbiage contains anything which is of the enemy. ["*Original*" cannot be overstressed here, because as can be seen; translating both *rhēma* and *lŏgŏs* merely as "word," is at best inadequate.]

It should not be overlooked that the definition of *lŏgŏs* also includes "something *said* (including the *thought*)...; "*reasoning* (the mental faculty) or *motive*...;" and "the Divine *Expression* (i.e. *Christ*)..."

Thus contained in the definition of lŏgŏs are the various aspects; both *material* and *immaterial*; to what may seem to be mere speech or merely "saying something." This seems to confirm the immaterial component of *any* action—here speech. The *action*; the *thought*, the *reason*, and the *motive*; are all components of the actuality. And as there are equal and opposite reactions for the material part; the same will necessarily occur for the immaterial components.

It must also again be noted that according to Strong, the use of "lŏgŏs" can also refer to: "the Divine

Expression (i.e. *Christ*)." Strong did not say Jesus; but rather: "i.e.," (Latin: *id est*), or "in other words:" "Christ." This "Divine Expression" (caps noted), thus does not likely refer to Jesus; who is *The* Christ (*the* Anointed One); but rather to *the* Christ or the Anointing itself; which of course refers to The *Holy Ghost* or Third part of the Trinity, and not to the Son, or Second part.

Thus this last part of the definition of lŏgŏs; the "Christ" or Holy Ghost part of lŏgŏs; seems to also describe a complete process such as: "Let there be light" and there was light. Again there is equal and opposite reactions as the result of the exercise of will.

Some of this "Word," (lŏgŏs), is contained in the Bible; most especially in The, (believed by many to be ten), Commandments. Some of this Word is in Science; some is in Mathematics; and some is found in Justice. In fact; wherever there is truth—therein is found the Word (lŏgŏs) of God.

Omniscience means that; among other things; there is nothing to learn. The enemy is not omniscient. [The temptation to state "in any way omniscient" is resisted here, as omniscience is a binary.] Ergo; the enemy can and does learn. When he encounters "judicial punishment" attacks via the "dirk or knife of the soul— which is 'the Word of God;'" he remembers to: "Be careful with that one. He's crazy. He 'knows what time it is,' and he fights back—and it hurts. I've still got the scars to prove it."

This will have a serious effect at the applied "voltage," forcing him to return at a more opportune time. It must remembered that in order to *return*, he must first *depart*. . . shall we say *retreat*?

———————————

The basic premise of Chiropractic; is that there is a Vital Life Force or "Innate Intelligence" which maintains the human body. According to Chiropractic, this force is 100% perfect; 100% of the time. It needs no help, but any interference results in disease, (dis-ease). There are analogous beliefs in acupuncture, and homeopathy—albeit each with different means of "remediation."

Chiropractic is concerned primarily with *material* interference to this VLF or Innate Intelligence. Thus; Chiropractors find levels of *material* interference to the expression of this *immaterial* intelligence, and remove this material interference. This material interference occurs *after* this immaterial intelligence enters the material realm of the body, and for Chiropractors, this is the nervous system.

As previously addressed, this intelligence is contained in this "breath of life" referenced in Genesis: *"and breathed into his nostrils the breath of life; and man became a living soul."*

Thus this VLF or Innate Intelligence originates in the *immaterial*, and by design is then received in the *material*; with its purpose being to maintain the material human vessel in a state of "health." When *material* interference occurs; such as in the nervous system by mechanical pressure; Chiropractors remove this material interference.

Years ago, Chiropractors had an interesting "joke," or perhaps a "ha-ha" would be a better description.

"*Subluxation Above Atlas*" was an intra-professional term that referred to various levels of mental insanity. This was generally stated in friendly manner. Since the atlas is the first vertebra, "Subluxation Above Atlas" referred to interference with that which was *above* the first vertebra, meaning a problem with the mental processes. [Practitioners of *craniopathy* excluded here.]

However; there may have been some degree of serendipitous wisdom in this term—

Is it such a certainty that interference with the VLF or Innate Intelligence can only take place in the *material* realm? *Material* things can interfere with the expression of the VLF or Innate Intelligence at the *material* level—but what about interference to this VLF occurring at the *immaterial* level?

Is there something in the immaterial realm that *would* or *could* benefit from causing *immaterial* interference to this immaterial VLF or Innate Intelligence in "hosts" (H. Sapiens); who according to the Bible; are by design, brought into existence primarily to wage war against said entity?

The answer to the "would" part of course is a resounding yes. After all what entity would not wish to decrease the productivity and longevity of *its* enemy? Surely there is ample motive.

But with regard to the "could" part, although this *seems* a bit more complex; in actuality only requires "connecting the dots" that have already been addressed.

Ask any competent physician: "When does sickness or disease occur?" The answer is when the external invasive forces overcome the internal resistive forces. Generally this involves the *material* realm: e.g.; invasive microorganisms. This can also be said of various types of physical trauma such as fractures.

This very same rule applies in the *immaterial* realm, as was previously addressed in Ohms law.

As previously stated:

> *"However; just as in Ohm's law, in order for this to work, there must be the load, and that load of course is the host. But being made in the image and likeness of God; that load (host) is not a particularly good conductor for the enemy's "current;" which necessarily means that the host is a particularly good resistor. In order to maximize the current flow for a given voltage; the enemy will also lower the host's resistance."*

It is important to understand the (true) actuality of "sin." The Greek word for "sin" often used in the New Testament is:

> "264 hamartanō; perh. from 1 (as a neg. particle) and the base of 3313; prop. to miss the mark (and so not share in the prize), i.e. (fig.) to err, esp. (mor.)..."[31]

The *reality* of sin, or that which is *perceived*; is generally limited to the action or inaction itself. However; again, it is the *actuality* of sin which truly exists, and "it is what it is;" independent of any limitations of *perception*, resulting in insufficient *reality*.

Here with *hamartanō*, we have the true twofold explanation of "sin." Not only is there error involved, but there is a subsequent and necessary *result* of this error. Here in this definition, the same being: "and so not share in the prize." The "and so" here reasonably meaning: "and so therefore because of this."

Thus this definition of *hamartanō*, tells us that the actuality of sin is twofold. Sin is not just the act of lying stealing, etc.; but rather both that portion and also the "and so therefore because of this." However; in this particular definition, to "not share in the prize," implies that a "zero" is possible. Meaning: that the consequence of sin could be merely to not obtain something of positive value. However this would necessarily require that there would be *no* "MA" for the "F;" no equal and opposite reactions; unless the "F" was positive in nature. Hence if this were true, one would reap what was sown if and only if it was positive; and reap nothing "no sharing in the prize" for negative actions.

Any and all actions, (and sometimes inactions); represent an actuality with two distinct but related components. The first being the *perceived* action; and the second being the, (secondary but necessary), *result(s)* of that action. Simply because the result is not contemplated matters little. One cannot have any action, without an equal and opposite reaction. Opposite here meaning: *towards* the source of the original action.

Thus; choosing the sinful behavior is always a matter of choosing the *twofold* actuality of sin; and not any erroneous *partial* perception—as ignorance of these laws changing nothing. When one chooses the actuality, one receives the actuality.

The laws of the universe care not one whit about any deficient perceptions. Sin is always a "package deal." Whatever behavior one chooses; one is also choosing and is bound to the *result*, as they are inextricably linked.

This is not to say that nothing can be done to mitigate any undesired result(s), as the creation of additional forces; e.g.; repentance, prayer for forgiveness, restitution etc.; can often mitigate circumstances. What is important to understand and remember; is that they *always* come together as a unit.

Following is a short excerpt from "*MeekRaker Beginnings. . .,*" Chapter 9: "*Job's Predicament.*"

"The following is likely the first great misconception which is purported to be in the Book of Job; as appearing in Job 1:8:

"The LORD said to Satan,
"Have you considered My servant Job?
For there is no one like him on the earth,
a blameless and upright man,
fearing God and turning away from evil."[MR1]

"In this passage, God appears to be offering up Job to the devil, and inquiring as to whether or not the devil would be interested in Job; this being precisely what many believe to in fact to be the case. But this really does not make any particular amount of sense. Firstly, God is not going to help the devil by suggesting or offering up Job. And secondly, an omniscient God would have known from the beginning of time what Satan's answer to this question was to be; as well as the very reason for which the devil was approaching Him at this time.

"In all fairness, it must be noted that some of the versions do contain a footnote to 1:8; which indicates that the original words that were correctly translated as "set thy heart on," were for some reason later supplanted by the word "considered."

"The *Interlinear Bible* confirms this: "Have you set your heart on" translation, as the correct translation of the original verse.[MR2]

"Now it is also fair to say, that the same argument as to why God asked Satan something that God already knew, can be raised with respect to the proper translation and understanding of this question. (And as though somehow Satan would actually tell God the truth.) In fact, the very same question is repeated, and again asked of the devil again in Job 2:3.[MR3] Of course God knew the answer to this question. It was not asked twice or even once because God was in need of this or any other type of information from Satan; neither is Satan known to be a reliable source for truth.

"The most reasonable explanation being that this was actually offered as a warning to the devil, in a question form. "Have you set your heart on my servant Job?" A more contemporary translation or translations being: "Are you really sure you want to do this?;" or; "Can I change your mind about doing this?," etc. Most people being given this type of warning by God would immediately reconsider. But not the devil, instead he starts complaining about how God is protecting Job etc.

"Job 1:9-12 tells us:

"Then Satan answered the LORD,
"Does Job fear God for nothing?
"Have You not made a hedge about
him and his house and all that
he has, on every side?

You have blessed the work of his
hands, and his possessions
have increased in the land.

But put forth Your hand now
and touch all that he has;
he will surely curse You to Your face."

Then the LORD said to Satan,
"Behold, all that he has is in your power,
only do not put forth your hand on him."
So Satan departed from
the presence of the LORD."[MR4]

40

"This represents classic Satan behavior. First he pollutes Job's mind with all of this doubt and subsequent fear. Then, after falling for Satan's meanderings, Job becomes terrified about the welfare of his sons, makes these continual burnt offerings; which establishes the f_t, and then Satan comes to God for permission to deliver the **ma**. And deliver this **ma** he did."[32] [Excerpt from: "*MeekRaker Beginnings...*" Chapter 9: "*Job's Predicament.*" © 2016 QPG, LLC All Rights Reserved. Reprinted by permission] [It must be noted that the lower case "f," rather than the upper case "F" was utilized. The use of the lower case represents the "force of *fear*."]

Here in Job, the enemy is instructed that all he (Job) *has* is in your, (the enemy's), *power*; but to "*not put forth your hand on him*," (Job). If it were the case that the enemy was generally *not* permitted to "*put forth your* (Satan's) *hand on*" a host; there would be little or no need for this instruction. Ergo; this ("*not put forth your hand on him*"), represents an *unusual* situation.

Thus; no other reasonable explanation exists other than the *usual* situation, is that Satan *is* in fact permitted to: "*put forth your* (his or Satan's) *hand*" on a host, as a result of said host's behavior.

How is it that an immaterial entity such as Satan; is in any way capable of putting his "*hand*" upon a material host, or anything material for that matter? Immaterial entities are not known for having any "hands." [Neither are *snakes*, (nachash), known to have legs or feet. But that is another matter. (see Genesis 3:14)]

It is interesting that Strong's provides no original Hebrew word for the word translated here as "hand" in verse 12—there simply is nothing listed. However the *Interlinear Bible* indicates that this word translated here as "hand" is: "3027 yâd."[33]

Strong's defines yâd as:

> "3027 yâd; a prim. word; a *hand* (the *open* one [indicating *power*, *means*, *direction*, etc.]. in distinction from 3079, the *closed* one)..."[34]

Therefore; the "unusuality" of this situation, is that Job is being protected from the usage of Satans's yâd; or his "power, means, (and) direction;" upon him *directly*. Instead Satan is only permitted to use the same only upon "*all that he has.*" *Indirect* attacks were okay here; but *direct* attacks were strictly forbidden.

Unlike the "normal" situation where Satan *is* permitted to "put on" or use his "hand" or "yâd... power, means, direction, etc.*" directly; here Job is being protected by God and God makes this quite clear to the enemy.

And we are or were told why earlier in Job 1:8: "*For there is no one like him on the earth, a blameless and upright man, fearing God and turning away from evil.*"

So unless one fits the above unique: "*for there is no one like him on the earth*" description of Job, one should not expect the same type of protection. Meaning: that the result of sin will likely be that Satan *is* permitted to "put on" or use his "hand;" (albeit an *open* and not a *closed* "hand"); or "yâd... p*ower, means, direction,* etc.;" *directly* upon us most, or at least some of the time. In a sense, here again the *actuality* of sin, includes the enemy having "permission to attack" or "judicial punishment;" as is also the case when attacking the *enemy.*

The universe respects the free will of H. Sapiens. When one chooses sin, the "sin" is always accompanied by the result [equal and opposite] of this sin. So it is understood that the "chooser" is in fact choosing the "undesired" result, as well and as the "desired" part of the "sin." [Again, "opposite" here in this usage, means *toward* the active party.]

As clearly seen in Job, behavior alters the *hedge* or *resistance* of H. Sapiens or hosts. And as previously seen in "Ohms law," and as seen with respect to *disease*; lowered resistance permits the entrance of undesirable and dangerous forces. Too low resistance in an electrical circuit permits an increased flow of electrons; which can damage or destroy the components. Too low *physical* resistance can permit the entrance of pathological microorganisms, which can damage or destroy the physical body. And too low a "*spiritual*" or "*immaterial*" resistance, can permit the entrance of the "hand" or "yâd... *power, means, direction,* etc." of the enemy—something from which Job was protected.

The enemy has the *motive.*

The enemy has the *means.*

What he or it *lacks* and is looking for; is the *opportunity.* And it is the lowered resistance or hedge; which is part of the "other side" of the actuality of sin; that provides him or it with this opportunity.

This is balance. The rules that apply with regard to attacking the enemy with the "the knife of the soul;" which is the *"Word of God"* in all of its forms; and even in a sense the "judicial punishment;" also apply to the enemy with respect to attacking H. Sapiens. The fact that most people simply "read over;" and therefore *miss* these *offensive* instructions *against* the enemy notwithstanding.

After all, if the enemy is subject to "judicial punishment" as the direct result of his choosing to act against the will of God; then this rule is the same for any other entity who chooses to act against the will of God. The main difference is that the enemy knows the rules, and collects. Those of "faith" generally do not know "the rules," and therefore generally do not collect. And often even those that do *know*, do not *understand* that this is *war*.

Satan means adversary; but this is only with respect to God; as despite Satan's wishes and beliefs; God cannot be killed. With respect to man however, the name "Satan" represents an understated term; as Satan can and in fact does cause the *physical*; (and he hopes also the *spiritual*); death of hosts. But Satan cannot ever do it alone.

God is about order and balance. Satan is about disorder and imbalance; i.e.; "creating chaos."

There are many types of "disorder" and "chaos" for which Satan is responsible. However the subject here is *immaterial* interference to the VLF or "Innate Intelligence," and the role of this interference in causing disease, and "premature" physical death.

If the "miracles" contained in the Bible are carefully analyzed, they fall into two categories: Those that actually violate natural law; and those that only *appear* to violate natural law. A miracle can only be a miracle—*if it violates natural law.*

With respect to the "miracles" of the "healing of the sick," the same is true. Again, the key difference is generally evidence of immediate physical changes. If a withered hand *instantaneously* is no longer withered; then this violates natural law and is a true miracle. However if disease is cured without any evidence of violation of natural law; then this represents not a miracle; but a matter of *authority* and *force*. And simply because this mechanism of "authority and force" is not known or understood; this does not necessarily or automatically cause the event to rise to the level of a true miracle.

This "authority and force," is merely the removal of the interference to the VLF. Once the interference is removed, then "normal" healing processes ensue.

It would be remiss to not address the following, which appears in Genesis 6:3.

Genesis 6:3 tells us:

> *And the LORD said, My spirit shall not always strive with man, for that he also is flesh: yet his days shall be an hundred and twenty years.*[35]

Two approaches can be taken with respect to this verse:

The first would be that this translation means precisely what it seems to say. Namely; that man is

supposed to live to one hundred and twenty years—
which is precisely how long Moses is believed to have
lived.

It must be noted however, that although this falls far
short of the lifespan of many of those in the early
Biblical passages; this, (120 years), represents an
increase in longevity of about 50% over today's average
lifespan.

The second approach would be that it means
something else. The same of course meaning; that this
translation, or the "common understanding" of this
translation, is less than accurate.

If this passage; Genesis 6:3; is examined in *context*;
i.e.; by examining the two verses *preceding* Genesis 6:3,
and the verse immediately *following* it; perhaps some
clarity can be obtained:

Genesis 6:1 tells us:

> *"And it came to pass,*
> *when men began to multiply*
> *on the face of the earth,*
> *and daughters were born unto them,"*[36]

Here in verse 1, is described what many would
consider as a "no-brainer." As man, (*"men"*), would
begin to *"multiply on the face of the earth,"* one would
reasonably expect that approximately 50% of this
"multiplication" would be female.

However; that, (the "no-brainer"), is not what the
passage is actually stating. Rather; this passage is
setting up the timeframe, or the "when" for the

introduction of an event described in the very next (Genesis 6:2) verse:

Genesis 6:2 then tells us what this event was:

> *"That the sons of God saw the daughters*
> *of men that they were fair;*
> *and they took them wives*
> *of all which they chose."*[37]

Here in verse 2, other participants are introduced into the event. These are in addition to the "*men*" and "*daughters*" referenced in verse 1—with this reference to the same now being these "*sons of God*." Here at this juncture; (the "set up" for the beginning of the previously cited verse 3); there are actually now *three* groups or classifications present. Here these are the original "*men*," the "*daughters*;" and now there are the "*sons of God*."

A clear distinction is being made here with respect to those who were *bearing* the "daughters," ("*men*" representing both genders of course); and these "*sons of God*" who "*took them wives of all which they chose*." Here it was not the "*daughters*" of the "*sons of God*" whom these "*sons of God*" were "taking;" but rather the "*daughters*" of "*men*."

Who were these "*sons of God*"?

The very next thing that follows these two verses, is the "120 year rule" from the aforementioned verse 3: "*And the LORD said, My spirit shall not always strive with man, for that he also is flesh: yet his days shall be an hundred and twenty years*."

47

The verse appearing *after* this "120 year rule" contained in Genesis 6:3, is Genesis 6:4; and provides some pertinent information.

Genesis 6:4 tells us:

> *"The Nephilim were on the earth*
> *in those days,*
> *and also afterward, when the sons of*
> *God came in to the daughters of men,*
> *and they bore children to them.*
> *Those were the mighty men who*
> *were of old, men of renown."*[38]

The following is an excerpt from "*MeekRaker Beginnings. . . Chapter 10: 'The Slanderer:'*"

> "This is a very interesting, but easily misread passage. Nephilim is the word: "5303 nephiyl, or nephil, from 5307; prop., a *feller*, i.e. a *bully* or *tyrant*: - giant. 5307 naphal, a prim. root; to *fall*, in a great variety of applications (intrans. or causat., lit. or fig.)..."[MR5]
>
> "The way this verse is normally interpreted, demons (fallen angels) had sexual relations with human women, and giants were the offspring of this union. These giants thus representing beings which were half human and half demon. This is the passage that is generally used to substantiate this theory.

"The problem with this theory; is that this passage in no way reasonably substantiates any such thing. It states that the Nephilim were on the earth already and afterwards, when the sons of God had sexual relations with daughters of men. It does not state when *they* (the Nephilum) had relations, but rather when the *Sons of God* had relations; thus making a distinction between the two. The "*them*" then referring to the Sons of God, to whom the children were born; and not the Nephilim.

"This demon theory also must presuppose that demons are to be considered "Sons of God." An argument would then logically follow that Messiah was the only begotten demon; which of course makes no sense. It also then follows that these Nephilim, half human half-demon beings are the ones who were of old and renown.

"An alternate read would be that the mention of the Nephilim is merely to state the relative time when the events of the rest of the verse occurred. Thus in this reading, the Nephilim were on the earth, but are otherwise unrelated to the remainder of the passage. It would then actually be those from the other side (the Hebrews) who were these Sons of God; who then had sexual relations with the gentile daughters, or daughters of the (gentile) men, and bore children to them; the children then being half gentile and half Hebrew."[39] [Excerpt

Thus it seems that these referenced "*sons of God,*" are or were those Hebrews; (ones from the "other side" of the *gan* or garden); the offspring of Adam, who (Adam), was *formed* by God from *something*, and not *created* from *nothing*—and within the past ten thousand years. These Hebrews were God's *chosen* people, because they were *chosen* for the bloodline for Messiah.

And these referenced "*men,*" are or were the offspring of those (the gentiles) who were *created* by God from *nothing*, perhaps hundreds of thousand of years ago.

Today "gentile" is synonymous with "non-Jewish," and in a certain very limited sense this can be true. However; the actual meaning of gentile refers to those "men" who were *created* and their offspring; such as the original *Chaldeans* who attacked Job; who lived on the earth long before, (and long after), the formation of Adam. This is why there is so much *Chaldean* in the Hebrew language.

Thus the "*man,*" (singular of "men"), referred to in Genesis 6:3 stated to have a lifespan of 120 years, is or are the *gentiles*; and not the "*sons of God*" or Hebrews.

Why is it that God seems to be playing favorites here? If it is assumed that being exempt from this "120 year rule" is simply a matter of genetics; then this would appear to be the case. After all, precisely how is it that one's parents are chosen?

However it is not a matter of *genetics*, but rather a matter of *knowledge*. It is *knowledge* of God's system, (and working within it), that increases longevity; and it is not merely a matter of one's ancestors. Through His Word one learns the system. And it was the Hebrews who at that time had this knowledge.

Perhaps a more modern translation of:

> *"And the LORD said, My spirit shall not always strive with man, for that he also is flesh: yet his days shall be an hundred and twenty years."*

> would be:

"I can only provide truth. If after 120 years of 'striving,' and they still insist on worshiping these false and dead "gods;" then that's it. I can only go so far in trying to get them to understand the rules, and it would be unfair and create a substantial imbalance to even try to do any more. After 120 years of being a hard head, (non-Meek— cannot be Raked); it "aint a gonna" soften."

Another view from a different perspective—

When the word *Kabbalah* in any of its various spellings is mentioned, generally ideas of some evil religion that should be avoided come to mind. The fact is that Kabbalah is actually not a "religion;" has nothing to do with "voodoo;" and simply means "*to receive.*"

It is true that Kabbalah professes many things that are inconsistent with Judeo/Christian tenets. The best example being the Kabbalistic view of Satan; which Kabbalists pronounce as "Suh-tan"—which is different from the Judeo/Christian pronunciation of "Say-tun." The Kabbalistic view seems to be that "Suh-tan" is actually deliberately provided as a means of human self-improvement.

This view is inconsistent with the Judeo/Christian belief that man was created in the image and likeness of God, and thus needs no improvement because of faulty design.

One might try to argue that this "image and likeness" is only the case in the first incarnation, and thus in subsequent incarnations improvements are required because faults are passed on with subsequent incarnations. Although this is clearly beyond the scope of this monograph; one would nevertheless be left asking the *cause* of the need for *any* improvements to a being *initially* created in the image and likeness of God. [See "*Reincarnation —A Reasonable Inquiry*"]

Thus either way; it seems that any need for improvement of H. Sapiens arises because of H. Sapien's succumbing to Satan's previous attacks. Satan is thus the *cause* of the need for improvement; and is *not* deliberately provided to assist in the correction of any "pre-existing conditions."

It is true that one can improve one's state by learning from one's mistakes—particularly as a result of the arrival of the "equal and opposite reaction" to sin. But without previous attacks; (as was the case with Adam for some period of time); there would simply be no need.

Nevertheless; the Kabbalistic concept of *Tikkune* merits some consideration. *Tikkune* is essentially the process of correcting one's faults.

It is unclear "Kabbalistically" whether *Tikkune* represents the correction of an individual's faults, or the discovery of an individual's true purpose in life; or both—meaning that the correction and the discovery of one's true purpose are two aspects of the same actuality. It is also unclear "Kabbalistically," as to whether said true purpose in life; according to Tikkune; represents anything beyond the correction of these personal faults.

If so; that is; that fault correction represents the true and only purpose of life; this also can conflict or not conflict with Judeo-Christian tenets. If it is supposed that the Bible is a book about *redemption*; which is something that is generally considered to be true; then one should reasonably and logically inquire as to precisely what it is that is to be redeemed.

If it is believed that it is only man himself that requires redemption; then this would be consistent with what this possible "true purpose" often suggested as the "true purpose" of Tikkune may represent. However; there seems to be no logical reason as to why God would have set up this type of system.

If however, the position is taken that redemption goes beyond personal redemption, and in fact includes the redemption of the earth; then things begin to make a bit more sense. But again, most erroneously believe that Genesis 1:2 merely represents a part of the *process* by which earth was created.

Genesis 1:2 tells us:

"And the earth was without form, and void;
and darkness **was** *upon the face*
of the deep.
And the Spirit of God moved
upon the face of the waters."[40]

However; there is a much more compelling argument that this is not so, and that the earth was actually completed at the end of Genesis 1:1—as after all, that is precisely what is stated. [see "*MeekRaker Beginnings . . .*" for irrefutable evidence in support of this position.]

Thus with this latter position, the redemptive process of the earth actually began in this second sentence of Genesis 1:2. At some unspecified time, God then created man as hosts or tsâbâ', to continue this redemptive process. This was due not to any lack in God's *capabilities*, but rather a matter of *authority*.

Tikkune is at a minimum, concerned with the removal of what Kabbalists call *Klipot*; or shells, rinds, husk's etc. According to Kabbalah, these Klipot block "the Light," or God.

If it can be stipulated that these Klipot are created as the result of behaviors inconsistent with will of God, and/or his rules; then these Klipot are created as a result of man's behavior. If it can be further stipulated, that these Klipot block "the Light" or God; then an interesting and pertinent illustration arises.

When Klipot are created because of what most would call "sinful behavior;" then there exists some blockage of "the Light" or God; including all of the emanations of

God; which necessarily includes the VLF or Innate Intelligence.

Thus although this VLF or Innate Intelligence is 100% perfect 100% of the time at the source of its immaterial *transmission*; these Klipot can interfere with its *reception* by the desired person. Thus the immaterial *reception* of these blocked or interfered with emissions is less than 100% perfect. Since these emissions are responsible for maintaining the health of the human physical vessel, the result would then necessarily be physical sickness, and/or physical death.

It must be asked as to whether this Tikkune process can remove currently existing Klipot; and if so whether or not *all* currently existing Klipot; and whether they are removed partially or completely; or if it is the case only future Klipot can be prevented. It must also be asked if any of this actually matters.

The reason why this might not actually matter, is that H. Sapiens are under constant *attack* by Say-tun, and are not being in any way directly or indirectly *assisted* by Suh-tan. In order to prevent *all* future Klipot, any given H. Sapien would have to immediately achieve *perfection* in behavior; which is essentially impossible when under constant attack, and in fact was only ever achieved by One. The same can be said for removing any existing Klipot. If there is a mechanism by which Tikkune could remove all currently existing Klipot; the same level of perfection would likely be required for sustaining the complete removal.

Thus at this juncture; physical life and death represents a binary; and physical death is a certainty; as any level of Klipot will block a corresponding amount of VLF or Innate Intelligence. And the result of any amount of VLF or Innate Intelligence blockage results is some degree of physical dysfunction, and thus ultimately physical death.

However; neither longevity nor physical health are a binary. The more upright the behavior, the fewer Klipot. The fewer Klipot; the less interference. The less interference, the greater the reception of the 100% VLF or Innate Intelligence. The greater the reception of the VLF or Innate Intelligence, the healthier one is, and the longer one lives.

———————

CONCLUSION

There is an immaterial world or realm. There must be. This is a necessity, from both the scientific and the "spiritual" viewpoints.

Science refers to the creation of the material universe, with said *process* commonly referred to as the "Big Bang" theory. The creation of the *material* universe necessarily represents an *effect* of something else. Science has no reasonable idea what that "something else" might be. That "something else" is of course necessarily the *cause* for the *effect* known as the creation of the material universe. [Just as an aside; this is where difficulties ultimately arise, as eventually there must be a *primium movens* or prime mover, or the *initial* cause. God is considered to be the causeless effect, which then caused everything else to be brought into existence. It seems that science currently has no plausible equivalent.]

Since the cause for this effect known as the creation of the universe: AKA: "The Big Bang;"" had to have existed *before* the manifestation of the effect; said *cause* had to reside *in*, and be delivered *from*, "somewhere." Since it could not have resided in the yet to be created material universe, it must have been "somewhere," other than the yet to be created material universe. Hobson's choice is that the source of this cause had to be an, or the, *immaterial* realm.

Even a Bible skeptic knows that the Bible tells us that God created the heavens and the earth. Where was God when He created the heavens and the earth? The answer is not stated. However as previously concluded; He could not have been in the material realm, ("the heavens and the earth"); until He created them ("the heavens and the earth"). Ergo; He was in, ("Who art in"), an or the *immaterial* realm, prior to the creation of the *material* realm.

As previously discussed, any time a decision is made to act or even sometimes to not act is brought into fruition, this represents two causes or imbalances. Thus there are two effects:

One effect is the balancing of the imbalance created in the *material* realm: "I threw the rock." Where the rock ended up is a simple material vector analysis. [A vector is a quantity with both magnitude and direction.] Thus as long as these factors are known, the rock's path and destination can be scientifically predicted. A spacecraft being sent to the moon, is essentially throwing a big rock—albeit with incredible force and precision.

The other effect is concerned with *why* one threw the rock. Depending on what the reason(s) is or are, different *causes* or *immaterial* imbalances are created. "I was mad and wanted to hit it in the head;" and "I had to stop that wild animal from attacking him;" represent entirely different causes. Thus even though the *material* forces might in fact be exactly the same; the imbalances created in the *immaterial* are entirely different. Thus the *effects* (equal and opposite reactions) of these created *causes* likewise will be entirely different.

Newton's "equal and opposite reactions," which apply in the *material*; also apply in the *immaterial*. This is sometimes referred to as *karma* or "reaping what one sowed." Jesus was advising on proper behavior, and not trying to provide analyses when he said to: "Do unto others as you would have them do unto you." The reason for this: is that whatever one does do unto others, will in fact ultimately also be done to him.

Here actions and reasons are being treated as two separate (material and immaterial) causes; but in fact they are actually one. Choosing to throw that rock in the material, includes also choosing, (as the result of the *reason*), the immaterial effects—effects which will ultimately; but not necessarily immediately; return to the material.

We are told that man is initially brought into existence in "the image and likeness of God." This can be represented by "A." This is not to say that this "image and likeness" represents in any way the *totality* of God; but rather that whatever man is when brought into existence, is entirely consistent with God. Man or "A" is a subset of that set which is known as "God."

Man may only represent a *partial* expression of God, but this partial expression is entirely consistent with the totality—for at least a nanosecond.

If it can be stipulated that the enemy wishes to change the "nature" of man, he must introduce these desired, (by the enemy), changes. These changes can be represented by "B."

What is this "B?" "B" is anything that is *not* consistent with this image and likeness of God. Thus "B" represents the *polar opposite* of anything that is in the image and likeness of God.

And just as man or "A" does not represent the *totality* of God; "B" rarely if ever can represent the opposite of the *totality* of mans portion of the "image and likeness" of God or "A." This is not because the enemy *would* not have this "B" be of the same magnitude as "A;" but simply and solely because he *cannot*, as opposed to "*will not*."

Thus it may *seem* that this could be expressed as "A - B = C;" with the resultant, or man's *condition* at any given time represented by "C."

However; given the actual circumstances it seems prudent to be better to always express this "B" in "A - B = C;" as "–A" to some extent in terms of *quality*, or *polarity*; but not in terms of *quantity*, or *magnitude.* Thus this: "A - B = C" equation does not hold; as: "A" – "-A" would in actuality be: "A" + "A." It is better understood as: "A + (-A) = C." This may seem unimportant, but it must be remembered that the enemy *introduces* factors that neutralize that which is of God.

Man spends very little time as "A." The overwhelming majority of the time man is "C." In fact for all practical purposes "A" can be ignored; and the status of man is "C." However this "C;" unlike a strictly numerical equation; retains any and all of the original "A" that was unchanged by the addition of "B, (–A)."

With the addition of "B," (or what is actually by design equal to "–A,"), to the original "A;" there is a "neutralization" of some of the magnitude of the original "A." This is what results in man's condition at any given time, or "C." If the enemy is able to add a negative; say neutralizing the "thou shall not steal" part of man, and the man is now a thief; this may not have any effect whatsoever upon the man telling a falsehood—although in many ways lying is in fact theft.

Neither is there any guaranteed permanency to the particulars of a given "C," at any given time. The thief may get arrested and punished, and not steal again. (Some of the best addiction counselors are former addicts.) Or a thief may steal a copy of this very Monograph, read it; and then understand that any perceived benefits from stealing are only temporary, and will ultimately be removed—likely with substantial interest charged.

This same "fluid" state exists with *immaterial* attacks on Innate Intelligence or the VLF. The actual percentage of the 100% perfect VLF *immaterially received* by man, (as opposed to reductions because of any subsequent VLF *material* interference); is a *variable* which depends upon how much of this "B" the enemy is able to introduce into the host, as per "Ohm's law."

Although it is essentially impossible to truly know, (science); or to truly understand, (wisdom); the immaterial realm—at least as of this writing; this nevertheless provides no license for not trying to derive some semblance of the processes, as well as the rules involved. Simply because something is not known or understood, in no way changes the fact that man must deal with the emanations from this realm—both "good" and "bad."

This *immaterial* interference to the VLF or Innate Intelligence likely occurs in two *direct* forms:

The *first* and easiest to visualize, would be the reduction of the amount of VLF received by the host. This would be analogous to, a simple blockage of the transmission, resulting in less than 100% reception of this force. This is similar to "closing the blinds," in order to reduce (block) the amount of light entering a room. This is similar to the *classical* explanation of *material* nerve interference by chiropractors. But chiropractors are concerned with *material* interference of this immaterial VLF, which is different than the *immaterial* interference under discussion.

The *second* direct form, would be to introduce *additional* emissions. Unlike a *blockage*, the creation of these additional emissions is like "jamming" a radio signal. The introduction of additional emissions produces errors; and likely produces them in two ways.

First is simply by the reception of these nonsense emissions. These are unnecessary and unwanted *additions* to the VLF which are simply nonsense; and thus disrupt the functioning of the VLF.

This is the *actual* belief of many chiropractors, in that in addition to *material* nerve interference *blocking* nerve impulses, *aberrant* impulses are created at the site of this mechanical impingement. But again, chiropractic is concerned with *material* interference, which is different than *immaterial* interference to the VLF.

And the *second* way these spurious "additional emissions" cause error; is likely the mixing of these nonsensical signals with both themselves and normal signals; (heterodyning); producing two *additional* signals; one equal to their sum and one equal to their difference.

There are three ways with which this *immaterial* interference to the VLF can be dealt:

The first is to do nothing. This is the predominant method, as here there is no general recognition of this *immaterial* VLF interference. Rather; the *material results* of this interference are "treated;" but unfortunately can only be treated up to a certain point.

The second is to modify the nature of these interfered with VLF signals at the site of reception. Meaning; that the VLF is modified by some type of "treatment" directly on or to the person. Homeopathy and Traditional Chinese Medicine [particularly Acupuncture, Moxibustion etc.] represent examples of this.

The main problem with the latter; (Traditional Chinese Medicine); is their current belief in "Deism" rather than "Theism." Since unlike Theism, which purports that there is an *active* God; Deism purports that although there is a God, He is currently not active. Why does this matter? Because without an active God, the *source* of the VLF is thus necessarily *internal*, or from within; rather than *external*, or from without. In fact; because of this change, that which used to be known as "Tao" was changed, and is now referred to as "Dao."

The third method is to remove the interference at its source. Christian Science touches upon this concept; however Christian Science is a *religion*. This is stated with no disrespect to religion in general, or Christian Science in the particular. But any religion represents a system; which although is generally formed based upon belief(s); is involved in many other activities and aspects of the lives of its members.

Modern day Christianity is almost exclusively involved with He who is the Anointed one, (Jesus); and not the *Anointing* Itself, (Christos), or the *source* of this anointing, (The Holy Ghost). "Christ" was not Jesus' last name. He is known as "The Christ," because of this Anointing—Jesus the Christ means Jesus the Anointed One.

The Holy Ghost, or the *third* part of The Trinity provided the Anointing to the Son, or the *second* part of the Trinity; with said anointing being known as "Christos." A fair read of The Book Acts shows that the concern at that time was in fact largely this "Christos" or anointing by the Holy Ghost or the third part of the Trinity, and *not* almost exclusively the Son—hence the name: "Acts."

Nevertheless; major religions today are grouped under a title, (Christianity); that was named such because of the capabilities of the Third part of the Trinity, and not the Second part of the Trinity; but are now almost exclusively concerned with the *Second* part of the Trinity, or the Son. This *inclusion* of the Son is both necessary and good. It is the virtual *exclusion* of the Holy Ghost that is the problem; as this, (Third Part) is where; even for Jesus, (Second Part); true miraculous power (dunamis) is found.

But how does one "remove the interference at its source?" In order to answer this question, a distinction must be made. There is a clear difference between *ectoparisitosis* or oppression; and *endoparisitosis* or possession—albeit with the point of transition often unclear.

Bacteria and demonic forces are both ubiquitous. In the material, if one is not careful, bacteria; being opportunistic entities; can and will *oppress* a host, creating a *parasitic* relationship between itself and the host. Meaning; that the bacteria will derive benefit at the expense of the host.

This parasitic relationship can be superficial and largely a nuisance, such as a small skin wound that has become "infected." Like with most battles, if the host engages in activities that the "parasite" does not like; this then begins a "reverse parasitic" relationship, in that the *host* is now acting in a manner believed to be to the benefit of the host and to the detriment of the bacteria. Keeping the area clean, and applying antiseptic will usually cause enough disturbances, that the tissue will heal faster than the invader can repair itself and its colony, or *nidus*. Here the microorganism is attacking from without, and is trying to get inside.

Or; this parasitic relationship can *increase* to the benefit of the invader with commensurate damage to the host. Impetigo, (from Latin *impetere* to attack),[41] is substantially more serious than "a small skin wound that has become infected," even though the same microorganism; *S. Aureus*; may be the "attacker." Here not always, but often; more serious and much more aggressive measures are required; including intervention by a third party, and often with the introduction of restricted chemical substances such as antibiotics. Here again the microorganism is attacking from without, but its "foot is in the door" and it is trying to get inside.

Once this or any other invading microorganism can truly get inside; i.e.; infectious systemic disease; matters change dramatically. At this juncture; unlike the previous two examples; the microorganism is now *within* and is attacking outward from within. Normally the VLF or Innate Intelligence is considered to operate "ADIO"—Above, Down, Inside, Out. Once infectious disease reaches a certain point, and subsequently begins to act from inside out; this can supplant the normal "IO" portion of "ADIO."

The first two examples above, represent material *ectoparisitosis* or oppression. The third example represents material *endoparisitosis* or possession— again, with the actual point of transition often unclear.

There are *immaterial* equivalents to the above three examples of material attack, or *impetere*. Just like bacteria, demonic forces attempt *ectoparisitosis*, or *oppression*, on an ongoing basis. As previously stated, it is when the external invasive forces overcome the internal resistive forces that sickness or disease occurs—both in the *material* and in the *immaterial*.

In the case of the *material*, these external invasive forces can increase simply as a matter of environment. Meaning; that if one spends time in an enclosed room with a large group of people who have contracted an infectious disease, the external invasive forces are dramatically increased. Thus it becomes quite likely that the normal internal resistive forces will be overcome, with the result being the "contraction" of this disease.

In the case of the *immaterial*, it is a bit different. As one behaves in a manner consistent with the Will of God; this will attract that which is *not* of God; e.g.; *demons*.

This may seem similar to the change of environment provided by the enclosed room full of sick people. However; here it is the case that the invasive forces are brought to the host, and it is not the host going to that environment.

However; as seen with Satan "complaining" to God about Job; there is simultaneously provided a "hedge" to protect this host. The nature of this hedge; (how high, how thick, how impenetrable); is determined by, and is the necessary result of, the balancing of the host's actions. *Materially*; this would be similar to a unexplained sudden increase in the internal resistive forces commensurate with the threat.

There is an interesting "side-effect" to this phenomenon. If it is so stipulated that there are a finite number of angels, and that the enemy took one third with him, (which is actually not true); then either way there are a finite number of these working for the enemy. To the extent that some of these are wasting their time "banging their heads" against a hedge, and likely complaining about it; they are incapable of mischief elsewhere. And even these mere *attempts*, set into motion forces that will return to them much to their dislike. The end result of this, is similar to an attack upon them.

Thus "upright" behavior necessarily results in increased demonic activity, with a concomitant increase in protection, (hedge), from that demonic activity. This results in the immediate and automatic provision of "Haz-Mat" protection. A host's resistance is not lowered, but raised. Again; this was the initial case with Job.

It is the willful engaging in "non-upright" behavior that then results in the provision of a "portal of entry," which permits successful immaterial *ectoparisitosis* or oppression, and/or *endoparisitosis* or possession. This *result* is not due to merely any increased demonic activity. And unlike upright behavior which raises the internal resistance; non-upright behavior lowers the resistance and thus this provides this portal.

Usually this portal of entry is provided because of emotional or *pyritic*; (Author's terminology, as iron pyrite known as "fool's gold."); decisions. These types of decisions are made because it "feels good" in the short term; with either no knowledge of equal and opposite reactions; or a transitory lack of concern, because it "feels good."

As long as the ectoparisitosis remains as such, a host's behavior can continue to alter the resistive portion; and thus things can change as a direct result of subsequent decisions regarding behavior.

However; just as is the case with material systemic diseases such as tuberculosis; once ectoparisitosis or oppression becomes *endoparisitosis*, or *possession*; this generally cannot be ameliorated or undone by the infected host. A discussion of this is beyond the scope of this monograph. [A rather exhaustive discussion of this phenomenon is contained in an upcoming new book—currently in post production.]

————————————

Years ago; in the attempt to obtain the utmost accuracy and precision; scientific weighing instruments were often enclosed in a vibration proof glass cabinet. These devices were such that they resembled the "Scales of Lady Justice," except that the two plates were supported from below not from above.

The weights to be placed on the one side were of such high precision, that if the tops of these weights were opened, tiny round spheres of metal were visible. The weights were cast slightly under the specifications, and these tiny spheres were then added for precision.

"Ms. X" decides she wants to make pound cake; [traditionally a pound of flour, a pound of butter, a pound of eggs, and a pound of sugar]. So to make sure it is "just right," she decides to use the aforementioned precise balance.

She places the highly precise and accurate one pound weight on the left, and begins to weigh the components on the right. However; when she weighs the sugar, she find out that she only has one half pound of sugar available. So she takes then a *half* pound weight, and places it on the left side, with the half pound of sugar on the right. And voila, there is perfect balance.

But she later discovers that no one seems to like the pound cake. This creates another imbalance, so she then convinces herself that the real problem must be that her guests must either be "gluten free;" or so "full" from the excellent meal, that they simply cannot eat any more.

Ms. X had (other) alternatives:

She could have simply made half of a pound cake, as here the sugar was the "limiting reagent." But then what would the guests have thought of her serving that tiny pound cake—that obviously was not enough to "go around?"

She could have borrowed a half pound of sugar from the neighbor next door; but then what could the neighbor possibly think of her then?

She could have gone to the market, but she was in the middle of cooking, and did not want to wait.

So instead; she did what "hosts" do on a regular basis. Huck Finn or Tom Sawyer would likely say that she "*let on*" that there was a pound of sugar; even though there was not.

The difference here being; that for children to "*let on*" that there are pirates in the cave, is necessary merely for the fun of the *process* of being children; and without any concern for the end *result*. But it is unclear precisely what end result it was that Ms. X expected, or could reasonably have expected; other than precisely what it was that happened.

"It all turned out for the best;" often results in both an *absolute* and a *relative* definition of "best." It is true that "best" is a superlative, and a superlative can neither be diminished nor augmented. "Almost best" or "better than best" are meaningless terms—despite any common usage.

"It all turned out for the best;" is usually stated as some sort of apology or acceptance of that which is less than "best." Ms. X might state this and provide some sort of justification(s) as to why this is so. But although the pound cake was better than it would have been had she used only one quarter pound of sugar, and thus when comparing the two, the disaster she baked was "better" than it could have been; it was only "best" if given only these two alternatives. This reminds one of when the former Soviet Union would lose a two team sports competition with the US. They would report the outcome as: "USSR came in second; and the US came in next to last."

The correct way to state "It all turned out for the best;" would be: "Given my ignorance, hardheadedness, stupidity, and belief that something is so simply because I say so—irrespective of what actually exists; it all tuned out as best as I would allow." Another might say that this actually represents one possible definition of "mercy."

When one chooses, one must choose from what is available. One cannot choose sin and not also choose the wages of sin. One cannot choose upright behavior and avoid the wages of upright behavior. Although the effects of the *immaterial* wages of sin have been removed by justification; *material* wages are very much alive, present, and quite active.

Understanding this, and acting in accord with this understanding; will allow, and arguably *force*, the "wages" of one's actions to be that which is beneficial— including a longer and healthier life.

ABOUT THE
MEEKRAKER SERIES

What on earth is a MeekRaker?

This word can be broken down into two parts "Meek" and "Raker." Capital letters were used in order to minimize any mispronunciations such as Mee-kraker; but the "etymology" is actually the fusion of these two words.

What is meek? And who in their right mind would ever want to be meek? Courage, strength, and bravery are characteristics that are generally considered desirable; but meek? No thanks. Unfortunately, the meaning of this word has been distorted over time to include things such as timidity, or shyness; weakness, or cowardice, but this is not; or rather should not be so.

Chambers states:

"meek adj. Probably before 1200 meok gentle, humble, in Ancrene Riwle; later mec (probably about 1200, in the *The Ormlum*); borrowed from a Scandanavian source (Compare Old Icelandic mjukr soft pliant gentle...."[AT-1]

These origins seem to be adjectival in nature, and describe a condition of humility or softness. Thus a meek person, by these definitions would indicate a humble or soft person. The opposite of this would then be a person who is prideful or hard.

Humble vs. prideful is an easy one. Who would want to be prideful? The Bible is replete with warnings about pride; and it was pride that started all of the messes to begin with. Pride may make one "feel good" for a short period of time, but as previously referenced; the Bible is quite clear that on that path there lies destruction.

But what does the Bible actually have to say about being a meek person?

- It tells us that the meek shall (*not will or might*) inherit the earth.[AT-2]
- It further tells us that the meek will be guided in judgment will be taught His way.[AT-3]
- The meek will be lifted up by the Lord, and He will cast the wicked down to the ground.[AT-4]
- He will save all the meek of the earth.[AT-5]

And what about the Bible's statements regarding being "hard?"

- "For their heart was hardened."[AT-6] "Have ye your heart yet hardened?"[AT-7]
- "... their eyes and hardened their heart."[AT-8]
- "But they and our fathers dealt proudly, and hardened their necks, and hearkened not to thy commandments, and refused to obey, neither were mindful of thy wonders that thou didst among them; but hardened their necks, and in their rebellion..."[AT-9]
- "Happy is the man that feareth always: But he that hardeneth his heart shall fall into mischief."[AT-10]
- "He that being often reproved hardeneth his neck, shall suddenly be destroyed, and that without remedy."[AT-11]

The actual word in all of these citations which is translated as hard is:

"4456 poroo (a kind of stone); to *petrify*, i.e. (fig.) to *indurate* (*render stupid* or *callous*): - blind, harden.[AT-12]

With respect to hard, there is a clear Scriptural relationship between the same and disobedience; not being "mindful" of God performing wonders in one's life, rebellious, falling into "mischief," and being "destroyed," "without remedy."

In addition, by the very definition of the original word, one who is "hard" is also stupid callous and blind. (If a physical heart were actually to turn into stone, you are just dead; so surely that definition does not apply in this context or usage.)

Thus, meek or soft; that being the opposite of hard; would tend to be obedient, be mindful of God performing wonders, not rebellious, not falling into mischief, and not destroyed. Furthermore, one would not be "stupid," "callous" or "blind."

The use of the term meek as "soft," also implies *teachable*.

Hardhead: will not change mind. Hardhearted: will not change heart. Hard necked: junction between head and heart is hard, and will not permit mental change to be transmitted to change the heart.

If it is firmly established that the term "revelation" has the prerequisite of being *the* truth; when confronted with potential revelation; it has been the authors' experiences that hard persons; specifically those of the head, neck, and heart variety; will generally behave according to the "Three A's:"

> A_1 is *anger*. This is the first response. This anger is not so much because there is a remote chance that they may be wrong, but rather when it is somewhat clear that they *are* wrong. This would be best illustrated as a line on a graph rising from left to right; with the level of anger represented by the vertical axis, and time represented by the horizontal axis.

A₂ is *argument*. This generally begins with emotionally (anger) driven arguments. As the arguments begin to fail, the level and usually the slope of **A₁** will increase. When all possible arguments, logical, relevant or otherwise have been proffered, the original arguments will then return. This would be best illustrated as a circle under the rising anger line referenced above. Often, what is just under the skin, (which is generally the reason for the pride and subsequent anger) will pop its "head" out; revealing things previously unknown about this individual.

A₃ is *absconding*. When all of the arguments and the repetition thereof have unquestionably failed, the hard person will generally abscond; or run away. This may be represented by actual physical separation, changing the subject or in some other manner. This could be perceived as the disappearance of the anger line, but is only subjective; as the true level of anger then becomes somewhat hidden.

Contrarily, the *meek* will weigh the value of any purported revelation; and then decide precisely what it is that merits their belief. Sincere questioning and even some arguments will be presented; but here not with the primary purpose of proving that they, the inquirer, is correct; but rather to understand precisely what it is that this revelation represents; knowing that if it in fact does represent revelation, then this will be to their benefit. A logical decision will then be made with respect to what constitutes the truth.

The primary basis for the actions of a "hard-head," is *emotional*. The primary basis for the actions of the meek; although perhaps including some emotional factors; (i.e. passion); is largely *intellectual*.

In a sense, the purpose of a rake is to separate the soft from the hard. The Bible refers to separating the wheat from the chaff, the silver from the dross; hence the origin of "*MeekRaker*". Meek or hard is not so much determined by what one believes; but rather by the *process* involved in making these determinations.

Bibliography

1) *King James Bible Romans 6:22-23*

2) *Strong, James. Strong's Exhaustive Concordance of the Bible. © 1890 James Strong, Madison, NJ p. 35 (Greek)*

3) *Strong, James. Strong's Exhaustive Concordance of the Bible. © 1890 James Strong, Madison, NJ p. 35 (Greek)*

4) *King James Bible Genesis 2:7*

5) *Strong, James. Strong's Exhaustive Concordance of the Bible. © 1890 James Strong, Madison, NJ p. 81 (Hebrew)*

6) *Strong, James. Strong's Exhaustive Concordance of the Bible. © 1890 James Strong, Madison, NJ p. 81 (Hebrew)*

7) *Strong, James. Strong's Exhaustive Concordance of the Bible. © 1890 James Strong, Madison, NJ p. 38 (Hebrew)*

8) *Strong, James. Strong's Exhaustive Concordance of the Bible. © 1890 James Strong, Madison, NJ p. 80 (Hebrew)*

9) *Strong, James. Strong's Exhaustive Concordance of the Bible. © 1890 James Strong, Madison, NJ p. 53 (Greek)*

10) *Strong, James. Strong's Exhaustive Concordance of the Bible. © 1890 James Strong, Madison, NJ p. 98 (Hebrew)*

11) *King James Bible Genesis 5:27*

12) *King James Bible Psalms 90:8-10*

13) *Strong, James. Strong's Exhaustive Concordance of the Bible. © 1890 James Strong, Madison, NJ p. 25 (Hebrew)*

14) *Strong, James. Strong's Exhaustive Concordance of the Bible. © 1890 James Strong, Madison, NJ p. 107 (Hebrew)*

15) *Strong, James. Strong's Exhaustive Concordance of the Bible. © 1890 James Strong, Madison, NJ p. 9 (Hebrew)*

16) *King James Bible Genesis 5:27 Deut. 34:7*

17) *Strong, James. Strong's Exhaustive Concordance of the Bible. © 1890 James Strong, Madison, NJ p. 27 (Greek)*

18) *King James Bible Proverbs 9:10-11*

19) *Strong, James. Strong's Exhaustive Concordance of the Bible. © 1890 James Strong, Madison, NJ p. 52 (Hebrew)*

20) *King James Bible, Exodus 20:12*

21) *King James Bible, Job 1:10*

22) *Strong, James. Strong's Exhaustive Concordance of the Bible. © 1890 James Strong, Madison, NJ p. 113 (Hebrew)*

23) *Strong, James. Strong's Exhaustive Concordance of the Bible. © 1890 James Strong, Madison, NJ p. 118 (Hebrew)*

24) *King James Bible, Ephesians 6:17*

25) *Strong, James. Strong's Exhaustive Concordance of the Bible. © 1890 James Strong, Madison, NJ p. 46 (Greek)*

26) *Strong, James. Strong's Exhaustive Concordance of the Bible. © 1890 James Strong, Madison, NJ p. 58 (Greek)*

27) *Strong, James. Strong's Exhaustive Concordance of the Bible. © 1890 James Strong, Madison, NJ p. 63 (Greek)*

28) *King James Bible, Ephesians 6:17 John 1:1*

29) *Strong, James. Strong's Exhaustive Concordance of the Bible. © 1890 James Strong, Madison, NJ p. 45 (Greek)*

30) *King James Bible, Ephesians 6:17 Matthew 4:11*

31) *Strong, James. Strong's Exhaustive Concordance of the Bible. © 1890 James Strong, Madison, NJ p. 10 (Greek)*

32) *New American Standard Bible: 1995 update. 1995 (Job 1:8) The Lockman Foundation: Lahabra, CA*

33) *Interlinear Bible Hebrew Greek English, 1 Volume Edition. © 1976, 1977, 1978, 1979, 1980, 1981, 1984. Second Edition,*

© *1986 Jay P. Green, Sr., Hendrickson Publishers (Job 1:8) p. 443*

34) *New American Standard Bible: 1995 update. 1995 (Job 2:3) The Lockman Foundation: Lahabra, CA*

35) *New American Standard Bible: 1995 update. 1995 (Job 1:9-12) The Lockman Foundation: Lahabra, CA*

36) *MeekRaker Beginnings..., © 2011 Quadrakoff Publications Group, LLC, Wilmington DE, p. 155-156*

37) *Interlinear Bible Hebrew Greek English, 1 Volume Edition. © 1976, 1977, 1978, 1979, 1980, 1981, 1984. Second Edition, © 1986 Jay P. Green, Sr., Hendrickson Publishers (Job 1:12) p. 443*

38) *Strong, James. Strong's Exhaustive Concordance of the Bible. © 1890 James Strong, Madison, NJ p. 47 (Hebrew)*

39) *King James Bible, Gen. 6:3*

40) *King James Bible, Gen. 6:1*

41) *King James Bible, Gen. 6:2*

42) *New American Standard Bible: 1995 update. 1995 (Gen. 6:4) The Lockman Foundation: Lahabra, CA*

43) *Strong, James. Strong's Exhaustive Concordance of the Bible. © 1890 James Strong, Madison, NJ p. 79 (Hebrew)*

44) *MeekRaker Beginnings..., © 2011 Quadrakoff Publications Group, LLC, Wilmington DE, p. 199-200*

45) *King James Bible, Gen. 1:2*

46) *Chambers Dictionary of Etymology. Copyright © 1988 The H. W. Wilson Company, New York, NY p. 512*

About the MeekRaker
Series Title

AT1 *Chambers Dictionary of Etymology*. Copyright © 1988
   The H. W. Wilson Company, New York, NY p.648
AT2 *www.kingjamesbibleonline.org* (KJV) (Matt.5:5)
   retrieved June 2011
AT3 *www.kingjamesbibleonline.org* (KJV) (Ps. 25:9)
   retrieved June 2011
AT4 *www.kingjamesbibleonline.org* (KJV) (Ps. 147:6)
   retrieved June 2011
AT5 *www.kingjamesbibleonline.org* (KJV) (Ps. 76:9)
   retrieved June 2011

AT6 *www.kingjamesbibleonline.org* (KJV) (Mark 6:52)
    retrieved June 2011
AT7 *www.kingjamesbibleonline.org* (KJV) (Mark 8:17)
    retrieved June 2011
AT8 *www.kingjamesbibleonline.org* (KJV) (John 12:40)
    retrieved June 2011
AT9 *www.kingjamesbibleonline.org* (KJV) (Neh. 9:16)
    retrieved June 2011
AT10 *www.kingjamesbibleonline.org* (KJV) (Prov. 28:14)
    retrieved June 2011
AT11 *www.kingjamesbibleonline.org* (KJV) (Prov. 29:1)
    retrieved June 2011
AT12 Strong, James. *Strong's Exhaustive Concordance of the Bible.* © 1890 James Strong, Madison, NJ p. 63 (Greek)

Other Fine QPG Publications:

MeekRaker Beginnings...

From the inside flap of "*MeekRaker Beginnings...*"

"The primary purpose of this tome, is the reconciliation of the word of God with science; and to do so in such a manner as to be rendered inarguable by any rational mind. As stated in the Preface: "One must choose between being a "man of science" or a believer," because they are generally considered to be mutually exclusive. If one agrees that words mean things, then an unbiased fair read of God's Word presents no such paradox. But one must read what God actually said, not merely what one thinks He said, what one was told He said, what one wished He said, or would rather He had said."

Wisdom Essentials—*The Pentalogy*

"That Which is Difficult If Not Impossible to Find Anywhere Else—All In One Volume. Vol. I"

But there are many other effects for which no material cause can be found. In "*Donald Trump*

Candidacy According to Matthew?," his meteoric rise and seeming inability to fail are explained according to Biblical principles. Since this is a non-political work, his success was not actually prophesied, but no other conclusion could possibly have been drawn—*and this was published long before he was even nominated.*

In "*SHÂMAR TO SHARIA*," the process of radical indoctrination is analyzed, and is shown to be a perversion of that very same thing God instructed man to do with the Commandments, and how this is not in any way limited to terrorists.

"*It's Not Just A Theory*" examines the relationship between behavior and longevity according to both science and the Scriptures; and "according to both" also includes major consistencies.

"*Calvary's Hidden Truths*" reveals many unknown facts about what actually occurred at that time.

"*Inevitable Balance*" scientifically and Biblically explains that which is often observed but rarely understood: Why "What Goes Around Comes Around;" AKA *karma*, or the "law of compensation."

STATISTS SAVING ONE

"The Malignant Sophistry of Rights Removal by the Far Left"

"...under the umbrella of "liberals" or "liberalism;" (as used today); there are actually two separate and distinct groups:

"True liberals believe very much in what they promulgate. They are truly concerned with the welfare of citizens, and they believe in policies that will benefit the same—at least in their view.   There are neither nefarious purposes, nor any intellectual dishonesty. Their objective is to improve the quality of life (and longevity), for as many people as possible.

"...Conservatives and liberals can often agree on the ends; but vastly disagree on the means. Giving a hungry person a fish is kind; but to conservatives, teaching him how to fish seems to be a better long term solution. It is not that conservatives object to the temporary giving of the fish; but rather they object to not teaching him how to fish.

"True liberals believe in the dignity of man; and promulgate policies in furtherance of this belief.
"Statists; the other group usually and often erroneously grouped under the "liberal" umbrella; are another matter. It is because of agreements with liberal policy that they are usually grouped under this liberal umbrella;

but their motivations, purposes and beliefs are entirely different—arguably antithetical—to true liberalism."

OSTIUM AB INFERNO
[*The Opening From Hell*]

"The Original Monograph - According to the Father, The Christ Son and The Holy Ghost"

"What is hell?

Why is there a hell?

What openings from "hell" exist?

What is the truth about "Abraham's Bosom?" And how does this or do these affect man?

What are angels? Are angels named such because of structure or function? Precisely why were some angels sent to hell? Is it true that one third were banished to hell? And when did this all happen?

Much of that which is fanciful has been written about these questions. But the answers should not be sought from that which is the product of men's imaginations—albeit these may provide interesting reading. Rather; the answers should be sought from, and always remain: "according to The Father, The Christ Son, and The Holy Ghost." (Written in English.)

REINCARNATION —A REASONABLE INQUIRY

"Often times it is emotion(s) and not facts that determine what it is that is believed to be 'in fact so.'"

"When truth and perceived practicality conflict; unfortunately it is truth that often becomes the sacrificial lamb."

"He that answereth a matter before he heareth it, it is folly and shame unto him."
                                                    —Proverbs 18:13 (KJV)

Some say reincarnation is a fact, and cite the Bible as the unimpeachable source regarding this matter. Others say reincarnation is fiction, and cite the Bible as the unimpeachable source regarding this very same matter.

One of these groups is about to be shocked.

QPG Publications are available
wherever you buy fine books.

95